Going Deeper: Angels and Dreams

Anna-Karen Sorensen

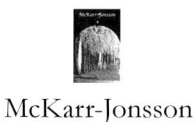

McKarr-Jonsson

Going Deeper: Angels and Dreams
Copyright © 2019 by Anna-Karen Sorensen

No part of this book may be reproduced
or modified in any form, including photocopying, recording, or by
any information storage and retrieval system without permission
in writing from the publisher.

Library of Congress Catalog-In-Publishing Data

Name: Sorensen, Anna-Karen
Title: Going Deeper: Angels and Dreams
Description: Book 2, Series, The Angelic Premie,
2019.
Identifiers: LCCN 2018912197 (print). 811.5
ISBN 9780980183030 (soft cover).
Subjects: Speculative Philosophy. Parents and
Infants. Pediatrics-Premature Infants. Psychology.

Design and Photography: AK Sorensen
Illustrations: Erica London Designs

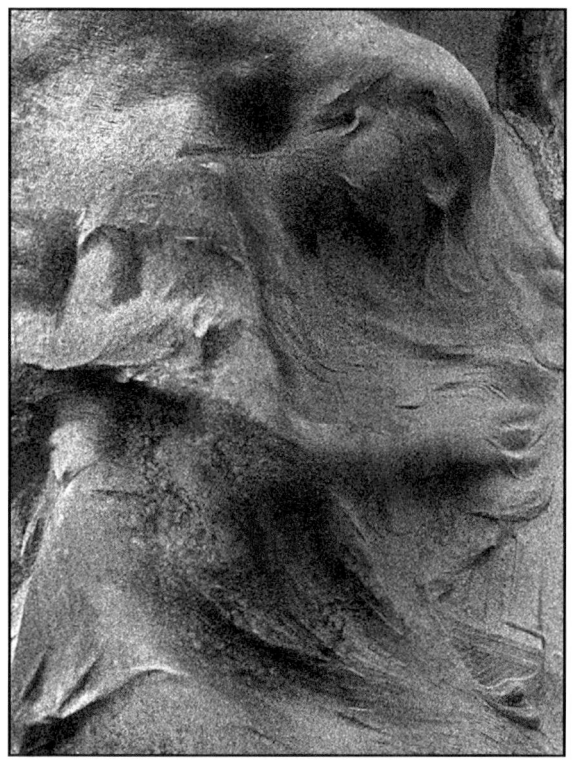

    A living work is a collaboration between the reader and the written word that jettisons something of the past into an ambivalent present in the guise of a reconditioned memory that recognizes its own Destiny. In this way, when the Time is right, something that was known but forgotten is rediscovered and Life's path adjusts its trajectory naturally.

A Fate Unwound Too Soon

Commentary

The subject of *A Fate Unwound Too Soon* is the too early born babe, seemingly in the world but not of it. The existence of the babe is not rational but irrational and ineffable, yet the senses are witnesses to it. The Mind reacts to the babe's presence becoming confused, seemingly threatened with a need to reconcile this perception with its own reality. It becomes plagued with a *dis-ease* that will not easily be put at ease.

The arrival of the too early born babe is powerful, filled with shock and awe. As an experience, it is different for each person who enters the infant's arena. Dealing with threat or loss is a unique process for each mourner and the Image that offers itself as an aid in this process is timely. Its form is dependent upon the relationship of the reader to her/his own Life. In order to allow for healing, each reader must enter the Symbol/Image at the appropriate point, taking the path that is best suited for a reweaving, which is to say, a mourning, burial and reclamation of an event so that it may enter Life again as an experience.

Table of Contents

Père Lachaise Image	1
Review *A Fate Unwound Too Soon*	2
Table of Contents	3
Preface	4
Image/Symbol and its Poesis	5
Spirit: Guardian Angel	9
The Angel	15
Art as Image	32
Axis Mundi	35
The Babe	36
Beauty Is…	39
The Body	44
Moving into the Body	53
The Carrier of the Idea	54
Consciousness	58
Death	67
Death Too Early	79
Truly Dead	85
Destiny	87
Divine	89
Doubt	91
Angels and Dreams	95
The Dream	97
Duality/Tension	104
Event/Experience	107
Fear	108
Idea/Eidos	109
Healing	110
Postface	112

Preface

The writing of the first book of this series, *A Fate Unwound Too Soon,* was a calling. The book just came together as a medley of what I had learned practicing medicine, studying the world psyche, and using light technically. I am asked why I wrote the book and what it means and I hesitate to explain for to explain a work of art is to strip it of its power.

Poetry, being symbolic, is embedded with the power to direct energy, but it becomes impotent, depleted of its wonderful energy if it is flattened by explanation. Image is describable and so I have, in writing this set of companion books to the original book, attempted to throw light on some of the many facets of the Images that carry the energy of *A Fate Unwound Too Soon.*

Image/Symbol and its Poesis

In this book, *Going Deeper: Angels and Dreams*, there is a discussion of Image in an expansive, multi-faceted manner, resulting in an empowering reinforcement of meaning through a slight shift in the use of words or phrases. As is true with the palimpsest, traces of one entry bleed into another investing both with a significance that surpasses the single layer/phrasing. In this way the reader is carried into a spiral of ever expanding familiarity with the Nature of the Images.

The words that chose themselves for this poetry are boundless. They took form within the rhythm of the heritage and were gestated within the meaning network of the culture. Poetic images carry both conscious and unconscious energy, residing as they do within a field of meaning that is shared by the Mind and the Heart. In this way, they are in the same moment both of this Time and untimely, personal and universal. Poetry initiates the process of healing, or becoming, with its ability to cross the bridge between what is known and what should be understood, carrying information between both states of being, closing the gap that keeps them apart and isolated from each other.

Raising consciousness for the particular as an individual or for the masses as a culture is the purpose of the Image whether it is Image as written word or as visual creation. As an exchange that is as particular as the moment and as vague as is required to accommodate readings and readers, the Image has infinite possibilities, much like Indra's net of jewels, every facet uniquely complete and yet infinitely interconnected.

> A Symbol does not disguise a thought, but reveals a Truth in its Time.

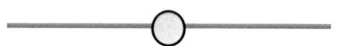

Within the movement of Love, as is true with Mourning, the connection between language and reality loosens as words become dissociated somewhat from the meaning understood by consciousness. Art is symbolic and so it has no fixed relationship with a field of meaning, rather it has a logic based on analogy that reconciles differences through recognition of likeness. In this way the Image/Symbol can speak in the language of the Heart to the Mind driven by the power of the movements initiated by the Angel, Love, and Mourning. It is with this fillip and energy that Life shifts its stance, taking the first step off of its plinth of Fate.

Poetry crosses the Mind's landscape riding on the wave of energy provided by its Images/Symbols. On the surface, poetry may appear to be something meant for the pleasure of the senses with its rhyme and rhythm, but it has the ability to move the goal posts to the advantage of Destiny. This comes not by soothing the senses, but by stirring the Mind with the power that is imbedded in Images. Poetry posits analogies that can hold tension and thus can muster and redirect energy as is needed.

Much of the dissatisfaction with Life, as a sense of meaninglessness, is caused by the distraction of ten thousand shiny things. Signs are mistaken for symbols and the old knowledge remains obscured by the numbing fascination with so much of so little import, overloading the sensory system with a sheer massive sameness. The senses are never free of vibration so that ears can hear the cooing of Nature and eyes can see the spark of the Divine emanating from within. Without contemplation the signs just keep glaring and blaring, reflecting off of the fluid surface of glassy eyes and the deafened eardrums plagued with tinnitus.

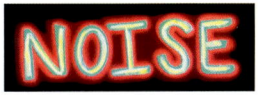

Without contemplation within the white of silence, the Symbol is misunderstood, or more correctly is simply understood, and is willfully thinned and placed safely within the already existent hierarchy as a sign.

Culture is the collective consciousness. Like the single Mind, it finds security in patterns and is less comfortable with change and the unknown. The greater the difference between the perceived reality and the irruption of the unknown, the more threatening the situation becomes and the more ill at ease the culture or the individual is. The threat of Death then, as the potential loss of all pattern and form, is the root metaphor for change and is the greatest threat of all. If the change is dealt with, transformed and given a name, then there can be entry into consciousness of something with meaning, an intuition that can lead to a Life better lived.

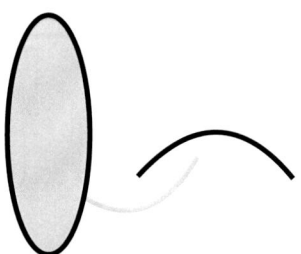

Spirit: Guardian Angel

The Angel is the image of the ineffable that being longed for will not let the landscape of the Mind settle. It is the Symbol that opens to both the Divine and the Natural, spanning the distance between what is known and what is forgotten, what is thought and what is not. A free spirit perpetually in mid-flight, the Angel is that which brings forth the unknown to be named and buries the labeled to be forgotten.

The Life force is the Spirit. Life begins with the sacrifice of the Angel who without wings deigns to tarry, a spark of the Divine, who with light footfall walks among us.

The Angel is uncanny, the strangely familiar that weaves its way through the fabric of the Mind. The wings of the Angel do not brush against the same branch twice for its energy is coiled and its trajectory spiral. It winds through the unknown yet familiar venues of the imagination to gather faerie dust for the enchantment of the Mind.

The Angel is the Image that yokes Reason to the irrational.

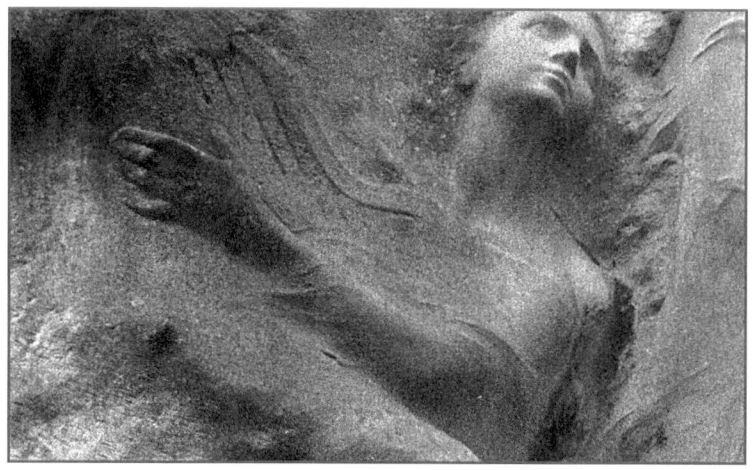

Père Lachaise, Paris

She is Plato's Spirit, an Angel
who brushing both worlds,
paint her wings with the colors of Life.

Spirit is that aspect of Divine energy that sacrifices autonomy to bind itself to the flesh. It is the guardian Angel that at all times remains conscious of the memory of the Original Vision as it attends to the business of Life.

The Angel is the Spirit which cannot be grasped.
She is the one who gazes at the Divine which cannot be seen.

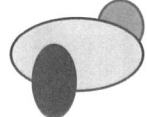

While the Heart is the seat of compassion, it is the Spirit that is the base of understanding. Being middle realms, both the Heart and the Spirit serve as interfaces between the perspective of Mind and the inclinations of Nature, the Heart using feeling and the Spirit Image as tools.

The Spirit remains connected to Nature through its native language, the Image, and to the Mind through Intuition. Being of two minds, the Spirit is reasonably irrational then, universal in an intimate way as it takes responsibility for guiding the Destiny of its charge. Through the Angel, the Spirit and Nature are connected, threaded together within the Image like pearls on a cosmic string.

Introducing Doubt as a thought, the Spirit causes the Mind to pause and take a second look at what it has treasured as belief. In the turn back that is the pause, the conscious Mind is rescued from its tendency to perseverate as it gives up the tired view, replacing it with the fresh Idea. In this way, Divine Wisdom becomes consciously significant as does thought become unconsciously relevant. Through the intent of Spirit, the unknown takes its place in Time and thought is given a footnote in Eternity.

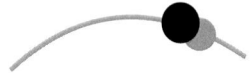

The Spirit, in its deep way of knowing, directs the restless energy of Nature and the feelings of the Heart into the Image which the Mind is then able to sense and to see. In this way, Spirit continually presents Ideas to the Mind, significant hints that are experienced as intuitions, which the Mind hopefully embraces.

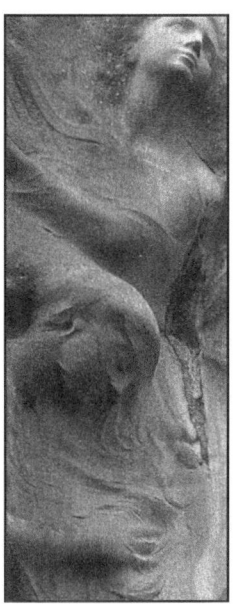

The Spirit is the spark of the Divine that is imbedded in the flesh of the Mind/Body as it enters Time. The Spirit is the Angel who is the guardian of the Destiny of the experiment that is the Life of the particular in the phenomenal world. In control of the direction of energy, the Spirit soothes the Mind, leading it to the whiteness of silence within pure prayer so it is relieved of the chatter and glare of the 10,000 shiny things. In this way, the Mind catches a glimpse of the Original Vision and carries it forward into Life. Through pure prayer, the Mind keeps the glimpse consciously close, warming itself with it, enabling the Divine to participate in the becoming that is recognized as the authentic Life.

The Spirit serves as the probe for the conscious Mind. Its energy is used to bring together in a congress, the rational Mind and the secret. Healing is sharing and the secret, in proportion, must be shared to consummate a cure.

> The view through the eyes of the Angel is colored
> by Life and lit by the Divine.

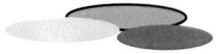

The babes as Angels stay with us for just a moment it seems; maybe it is longer, but they all pass through. Some set anchor in Time, but others never cut the tether to the other world. Either way, they touch us and we are renewed by it as they leave their traces upon us, a bit of something Divine, fairy footprints upon the moist pastures of our memory.

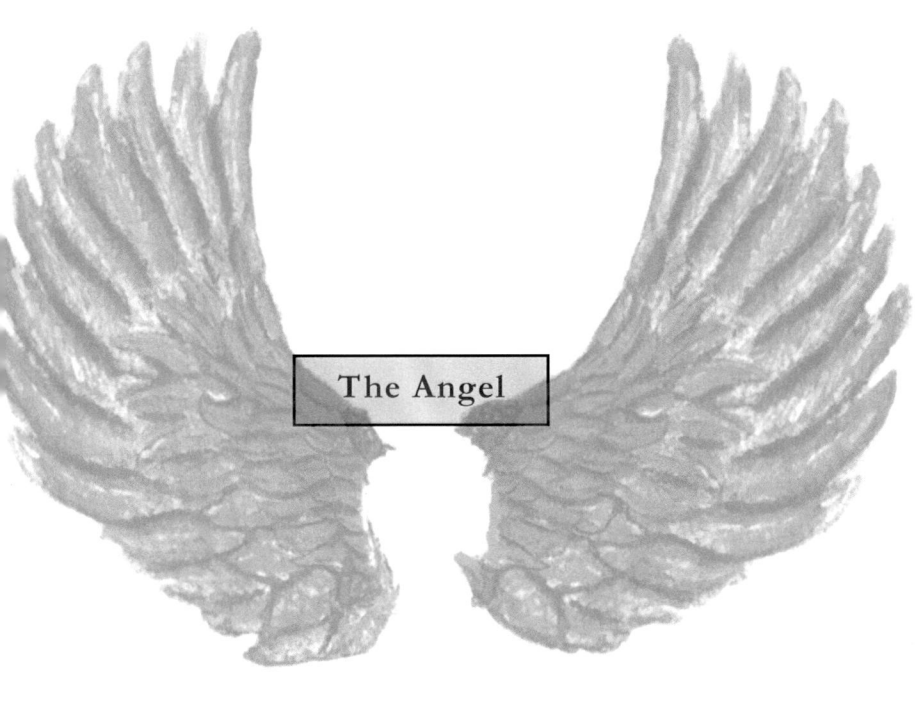

The Angel

With every breath of the babe,
an Angel sighs.

> The Angel directs energy.
> It is the carrier of the Idea from the
> Pansophy.
> It is older than memory and newer than Life,
> as it comes Into Time.

The Angel is both figurative and literal, loved and longed for, and she will not let the Mind rest. Her energy is coiled, not the straight line that leads to the past and future of Time. Nor is it the cyclical rumination that leads to mere repetition. She is strange and yet also familiar. Having forgotten that we knew her, we follow her instinctively and long for her, anticipating revelation.

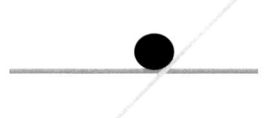

What Angel Is This

What angel is this
Who losing its way
Falls into the Time
Of my Life.

Falls out of its world
and into my spring,
a flower to color it in.

To fill in the outlines of
my thought balloons
with the hues and shades
of Light.

So the empty cartoon,
My series of events,
becomes an evocation
beckoning Life.

By the Hand of the Angel

The Angel walks us deep
Into the forest of the Mind
But only as far as she can see
In the dimmed down glow of Time.

The trees grow longer shadows
Virgins cast sharp in her light
And the crooks of the bark
Appear ready for a fight.

The Angel as psychopomp
With warm heart, hand so cold
Pulls hard against resistance
Accompanying the old.

Who weighted as though chained to Time
Are pulled against their will
Grasping all familiar road signs
Of the world they long for still.

But with the last grasp broken
The anemic fades from view
And that which lived before today
Is inspirited anew.

By the agency of the angelic realm,
what is recovered carries the
fragrance of newness as
well as the scent of
familiarity.

The Angel creates a rent in the veil that separates her world
from Time, so that we might feel the breeze from her beating
wings and follow her back to our roots.

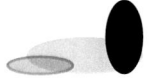

Breeding parthenogenetically, the Angel initiates its
own movement, investing in
itself.

Blithe spirit

The littlest Spirit
So light it needs no wings
To fly into the chambers of my heart.

The Angel breaks the endless cycle, the tachyphylaxis that comes with Mindless repetition.

Like the surge of the sea, the Angel always comes
and like the sea she withdraws again,
leaving behind pearls,
intuitions housed in familiar shells.

Tip toeing through the heather of Nature, the Angel sets out on its journey and in so doing, sends a shiver up the spine as it quickens the pulse and sets the Mind to quivering.

Into Life

Like a fledgling fallen
heavily from the nest,
the Angel lies anchored by weight.

Who once was so light,
is now heavy with flesh,
its Nature encased in skin.

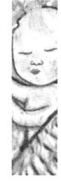

The frame of the feathered wings,
articulated with such grace,
appear now as boney stumps.

Its clairvoyance fogged in,
the Angel's horizons dim
to the scan of its Mind's eye.

So, the babe lies before me,
blind and breathlessly mute
as the Truth is secreted away.

Coming into the vexation
known as Time and Space
where Truth will have to be sought.

The Angel presents a bouquet of the forgotten
somethings that were at one Time embraced as personal, now lost
to Time.

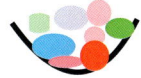

Being both literal and figurative,
the Angel vacillates between the real and the imaginal realms in
order to tutor the Mind in
unpleasant Truths.

We cannot capture the Angel intellectually. We can only sense its presence when we look down upon the porcelain body of the being who is present among us, but is not yet committed. We see a creature who is unnatural and outside of the normal rhythm of Time and we are filled with awe, our Minds are stilled, and for an instant we glimpse the Divine.

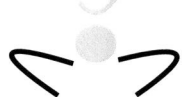

The Angel exists in the in-between.
It is not conceived of consciously,
but is an energy bearing Symbol necessary to move between
the two ways of being in the world,
thinking and knowing.

Moving between the world as sensed and the world as intuited,
the Angel lights, having carried the question away,
it returns with a reply.

●

The Angel, once flesh of the imagination,
now born into Time as the beloved,
the tiny babe.

●

The Angel leaves marks of her having been here for us to
follow home,
breadcrumbs back to God's house.

Life saccades along a thread of conscious events leaving the impression of a memory sequence with one thing seeming to occur after another in a fairly predictable pattern. Daily Life has few deviations which, if there are any, are for the most part handled by the conscious censor. But when the babe lies near us, just near enough for us to listen to it breathe, the clicking of seconds attenuates and we slip behind silence, hovering within Time as we waft past the edges of Being. As with Quantum's nonlocal event, within the experience of the too early born, all can be felt and known instantly as the conscious Mind goes to sleep and the imagination comes out to play.

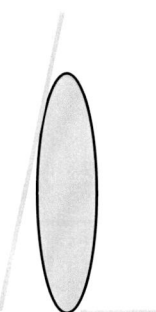

In the night, the Angel is the image that haunts the Dream,
becoming on the following day the figure on the street
that pulls the attention.

The Angel suspends itself between harmony and disharmony, the Wisdom of the Divine and the Knowledge of Nature, feathering its own reality. As Spirit, it is beyond the control of consciousness as it energizes its own movement, investing it itself. Twisting back and relaxing forward, gazing upwards and reaching down, it rescues a Truth. Something enters into consciousness and nothing will be the same again. As Spirit, the Angel leads us back to ourselves.

We catch but a glimpse, a hint that there is something beyond
consciousness that is evermore available,
a *suchness* to be longed for.

The Angel leaves a scent that beckons
consciousness towards its own Nature.

Porcelain Angel

Porcelain angel who so doll like
Pillow-wings behind her head
Lies iridescent in divine Light
Its white silence o'er her bed.

Only God can see her this way,
And the Angels who gaze ahead
Along a beam of Heaven's Light
To the babe in infrared.

Infrared is light of a wavelength that is not perceived by the human eye. Infrared film reacts chemically with the energy that comes from the body of the babe, so that on the negative we capture some of the essence of the enfleshing Angel.

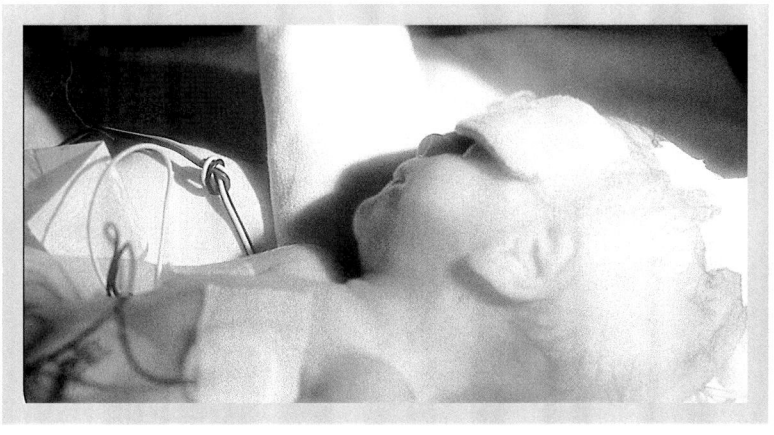

The babe as Angel, comes directly from the side of the
Divine, from the place of the silence of white.
Its memory of the Original Vision is pure,
but with Time it becomes dusted with the pollen of
Nature. Thus veiled,
the Angel as babe can do little more than intuit.

The experience of the babe is liminal. A sense of it inhabits the Mind, leading it to hear, to see, and to know against the natural grain of consciousness which is designed to filter, to exclude, and to willfully redirect energy so that it can preserve what it understands. The babe being quite beyond understanding and yet an intimate, steals into the Mind, imploring it to deal with the newness of its reality.

The conundrum caused by the arrival of the babe in the moment that is right, but not convenient, necessitates that there be an adjustment in perspective, and thus some discomfort. The power of the angelic movement, put into motion by the arrival of the babe, energizes the event as it shape shifts into an experience. The significance and the rightful inclusion of the other becomes more apparent and the natural tendency of consciousness to exclude is overwhelmed by compassion as the other is given room in the Heart and Wisdom is given permission to rise and rest next to the cradle.

The Angel as Spirit initiates its own movement. It leads us to twist back in the unnatural motion of reflection that requires an uneasy intimacy with the unknown, a recalling through the distortions of memory. In this way, the beloved is brought back to Life, not as it was, for it is different and is seen differently. The beloved is now its true self, not what was longed for, but what is needed.

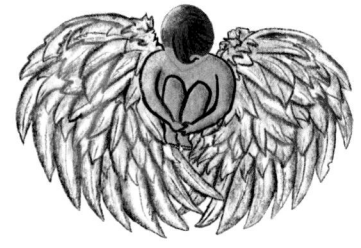

The Angel who in Life is just a bit too far away, becomes in
Death an intimate, unreasonably close so that what was once
comfortably placed without comes to reside
uneasily within.

Art as Image

Art demands something of the witness; the eye must gaze to see or the ear must listen to hear. It is the deeper Wisdom that screams to us from the screen, from the page, or from the song. With Art, we let go of expectation and allow ourselves to be surprised, gifting ourselves with thought-free space for the question that needs to be asked to come to Mind.

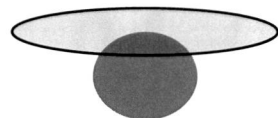

Art is a mural upon which the unconscious is projected in all of its multifarious wonder. It is a liminal space where consciousness is held in suspension as the world as lived and the world as imagined meld within one language.

Serving as a stand-in for the Mind/Body, Art is a depiction.
It is an exteriorization of the Dream of the auteur as she/he gives
freedom to a Truth that had been reduced to a belief,
a Truth imprisoned in Time.

Art induces the movement of energy from the particular to the
general, from the psychic space of an individual
to the consciousness of the culture.
Art speaks with the logic of humanity
in the voice of one being.

Art leaps across the vistas of the Mind and the breadth of the
culture; it minimizes the distance between what is and
what could be.

The repeated use of an Image, or iterations of it, increases its potency and the likelihood that a change will be brought about in the psyche of the individual within a culture and as a result, to the social matrix. When the variant shadings of an Idea are summed, they become part of the world we know as it morphs into the world that we imagine it to be. This is the power of the Image as Symbol when it speaks to an audience at the right Time and in the right way; it brings to Mind the questions that have remained unasked.

Axis mundi

The babe is the center of this world, one could say the *axis mundi* of *A Fate Unwound Too Soon*. It initiates a movement, snagging the chosen ones as it entangles them in its narrative, taking what was someone else's story and transforming it into a personal myth. The babe, as Angel, takes the wasteland that living can become and imbues it with authenticity again.

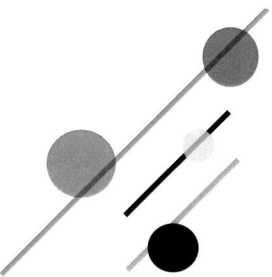

The Babe

The Babe is the Angel who, as the Image of the ineffable, becomes personal within Time.

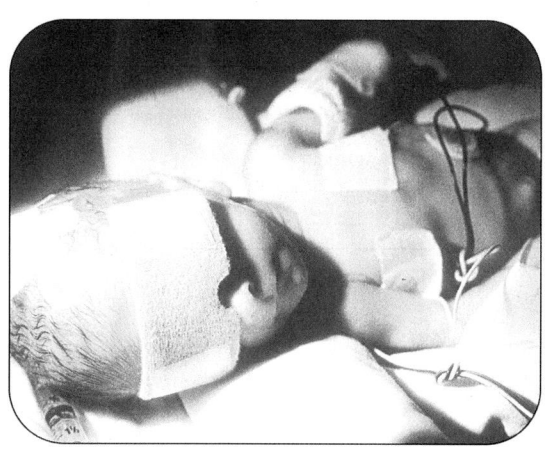

Flowers live in Time, so they have but a moment. Fragile like the babe, their pedals bruise easily and their stems break with carelessness. Like the babe, they list toward Death as soon as their connection to the source is severed. The tiny babe, like the bud of the flower, is a manifestation of the Divine, a thing of Beauty hiding its colors within.

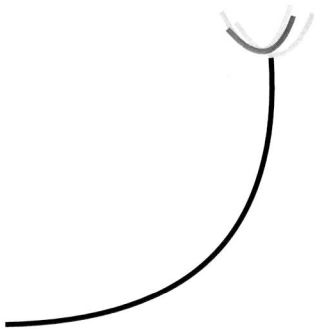

The babe is the Angel who pulls our attention towards it, lulling our Minds and awakening our Hearts to its Beauty. Being near enough to feel it live, we fall out of our world and under its spell. Crossing the distance between what is and what might be in the moment of the glance, we, like the heliotrope, bend our faces towards its divinity, arcing Eternity.

> The Beauty of the babe, the awe-full Nature of it,
> startles the imagination, filliping the psyche to move beyond
> what is understood,
> to what is not.

The authentic Life is salvaged with the arrival of the babe. The experience of its Nature is the means by which the loved ones and caretakers make their way back from the state of amnesia that plagues humanity today. Whether the babe decides to stay or choses to leave and return to the side of the Divine, it draws those near to it into its crisis and gifts them with a glimpse, a split second of an unsettling energy that must be handled. This overpowering energy must be processed and given some of the character of consciousness so that what was meant to be brought to light can be intuited.

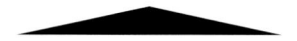

> In the presence of the too early born,
> we share a moment outside of Time
> with something risen from the marrow,
> with something that we know instantly and deeply has to do
> with all that ever was and will be.

Beauty is ...

Beauty is value that is measured,
so is it relative or absolute?
It is both, as the Ideal and its emanation, the Beauty that is
shared by all things.

"Real Life (which is the presence with the divinity) is
actualization of intelligence…thereby begetting beauty…"
(Plotinus VI.9)

Beauty is to be found everywhere.
Good is in everything.

Beauty is experienced as the revelation of the concealment,
the Divine hidden and revealed.

Beauty is incomprehensible; it is a way of knowing that cannot be articulated and a way of being that the saccade of the Mind's eye fails to catch. Being independent of context, Beauty is the Good that lies within all things at all times, the eternal oneness that is experienced as sympathy.

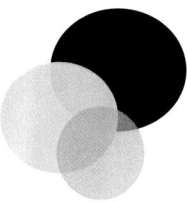

Beauty is the felt reaction to the glimpse of Divine radiance which startles the Mind and wakens the imagination. Even in its absence, Beauty provokes movement toward it as yearning replaces awe. Like the luster that winks, Beauty is suggestive, fostering an intimacy that initiates the desire to share.

To sense the Angel is to be conscious of the Beauty
that is within.

There is a silence in white, a unity, which when fractured by the prism, becomes a rainbow, a plethora of hues and shades to color the earth and fill its Time with Beauty. Adorned with the essence of the Divine, Nature is painted across Time as the flowers of the fields.

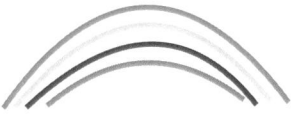

Beauty is a theophany.
It is that catch in the peripheral vision of the Mind's eye
that leaves its trace on the retina,
an aura portending potentiality.

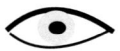

Beauty is universal and is not dependent upon context.
The reaction to it is immediate
and cannot be reduced to words of description.
It is the sense of the presence of an Angel,
a knowing that cannot be articulated.

Beauty is suggestive and is capable of stirring the imagination,
providing the impulse to *un-forget* in a selective
remembering of the unknown.

So the babe enters as a manifestation of Beauty.
It solicits a movement away,
a shifting toward the Good.

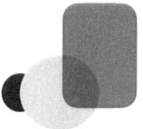

The promise that is Beauty,
like the babe,
offers but a glimpse before it fades away.

The Heart feeds on the Beauty of the Spirit.
The Mind starves for lack of it.

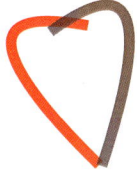

Like the Angel,
Beauty that is born of compassion is the *a priori* secret,
the luster that fosters intimacy, tearing down the walls of the
intellectual sanctuary.

The Body

The Body is the subject of experience. It is the membrane through which the information of reality is exchanged for the Ideas of the imagination. It is the means by which the Divine gains experience of the world. The conscious Mind, growing ever wider and deeper, gains knowledge of its own creator, not by living on the surface, distracted by ten thousand things, but by moving behind thought and fear to discover the Divine Nature within.

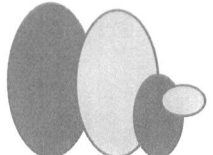

Let me have the sense of you,
since Body I could not
and curl up in my empty Heart
its walls a swaddling cot.

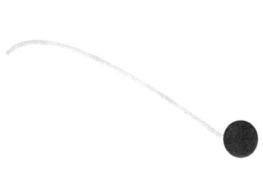

The Spirit naturally extends into Space.
It is the Body that tethers it to the earth.

Amnesia of the Truth is the plague of the human race.

Outside of Life, the Spirit is free to soar, but enfleshed, its entrapment is experienced by the Body as symptom, by the Heart as feeling, and by the psyche as intuition. The Body needs to be recognized and honored. It needs to be brought into the conversation and its Wisdom, imbedded in the genetics of inheritance and the experiences of humanity, should be embraced. Without giving place to the needs of the Body, its energy becomes a tyrant longing to push someone around.

> Through the Body,
> one participates in the world.
> Through the rooted Mind, one participates in Life.

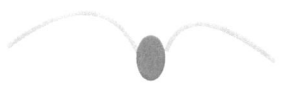

The Spirit sets itself to the pace of Time so that the Divine has some presence in Life.

Living Life as a daily cycle of consciousness gives voice to a persistent soughing, a whisper that calls longingly for something that is missing. This something is the Body, the vessel through which Life comes into being. Anesthesia to the body allows the Mind in its isolation to maintain an elitist posture, keeping its own company. The intellect as the power to rationalize becomes walled off from the experience of feeling and the blessing of knowing.

The dissociation from the Body in the West, which began in earnest with Plato and became exaggerated after Descartes, has been the source of an alienation experienced as a sense of absence. To rescue the Body requires a flight from Descartes and the paranoia of the talents of the flesh and a return Nature and the healing gnosis of the Body.

The Body of the Mother
The Body of the Babe

I stand, a pillar in the midst of a storm,
just a member of the cast.
Set in a cloud of doubt, no longer with any clout,
what role do I play?

Then the eye of the squall passes over the stage
and for just a moment I can see
that the scene has changed and what God has arranged,
is no longer intimate to me.

The babe had become "Borg,"
what was once, one with my flesh
is now corded to machines.

So I withdraw to my place,
to my own proper space
to wait for the eye to move on,
for the storm to resurge in a swirl of acts
as I wait for the end of the play.

The Body is the interface though which one perceives events and gains experience of the world. One must move beyond the immediately given. That is to say, one must move deeper into an event, transforming it into an experience. If one remains on the surface, the event remains just another distraction with which the world is replete.

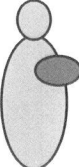

When cultures cut themselves free of Nature,
they lose the talent to appreciate the subtle perceptions
of a beautifully muted world.

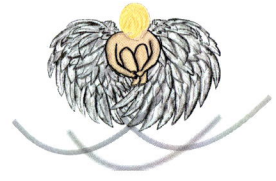

"A Crack in the Garden Wall"
Birth into Life Through the Body

In Heaven: No thorn to prick the finger
No blood red drops to fall
No stain on the snow of innocence
No fragrance to bring one to sad memories
No hindrances to the knowing of things.

At Birth: And then the gate opens just a bit,
just enough for the smallest Angel to pass through.
Her eyes open wide as she looks ahead.

She feels herself pulled toward the crack.
She can smell the must of the otherworld,
of Life wafting towards her.
She hesitates for she understands the sacrifice.

But the opening is for her.
It is her moment
or more correctly,
it is the Time for her to leave.

She knows it is inconvenient
and there can be no turning back,
so she fills her little Angel lungs
with one last breath of heaven and steps away
from the safety of white.

Reality: For all of the Beauty of the garden,
even with its perfection,
Necessity called and
she was drawn to another way of being.

Carried inward by the Angel, Love or Mourning, the Mind moves closer to the natural realm where consciousness, isolated as it tends to be, can find its connection to the earth and to the Body again. The Body when alienated from the Spirit, is Mindless and thus deprived of the nourishment that is needed for the root to grow along its natural path.

The Earth is the dust of which the Body is made, the field on which the game of Life is played and the repository to which all is returned. The Body is a footprint that dissipates as Nature exhales. Begun in moisture, in the darkness of her, the Body ends as a desiccation, a dry leaf blown away from its tree.

Moving into the Body

There is a timely process by which the Spirit is enfleshed, but with the premature birth, the embodiment is expedited. There is urgency, then the appearance followed by silence. Ambivalence arrives as the babe brushes both worlds with her wings, turning back to the unknown, hesitating in a moment of doubt.

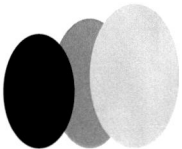

The greatest sacrifice for an Angel to make is
to step down into Life.

The Carrier of the Idea
The Chosen One

The chosen one is the one who makes a difference. A living entity which acts as a transformer, as a Symbol which redirects energy.

Detaching from the universal and becoming unique,
the chosen one is a child of Destiny
whose original thinking and daring departure from the collective offers the wonderful gift of surprise to the world.

The chosen one understands and is comfortable
with the Truth of the unknown. She/he leads us into the
forest without fear.

The carrier of the Idea is the one who walks between, reinforc-
ing the paradox so there is always potential for change.

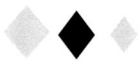

The babe is the Wisdom of the Divine become flesh,
the Carrier of the Idea for those who would learn.

A Chosen One

Arising out of the irrational
At the behest of necessity
Is a wished for child, a chosen one
To bring us round to see.

The Angel is both active and passive, the carrier of the Idea and the message in understandable form. It reminds us of what we knew but forgot we knew before the veil of Time was drawn across the memory of our Minds.

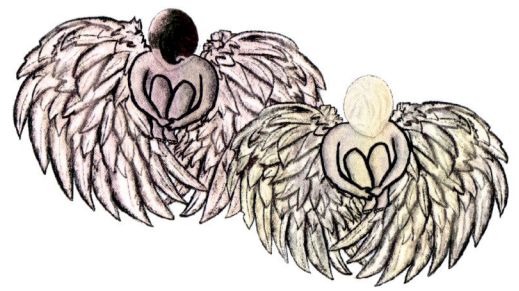

Each New One

Each new one is a powerful thing.
Awed, we gaze down upon it,
a wonder more unusual than most,
the babe is a lesson just as it is.

The Babe is the hope of the world,
the one who will tear down the standard
around which the culture has gathered,
shredding it with the sharp edge of an Idea.

All is possible for the Carrier of the Idea.
While we are tired, conservative, cautious,
the new one is without constraint,
for she contains unbounded potential.

Not having the learned lessons of Life,
the Chosen One still feels the source;
he is not yet constrained by
the resolve to follow one path.

In the new one lies the rescue
of the many and the one
if they are so inclined to receive her
as the Carrier of the Idea.

Consciousness

As with the cut flower, the Symbol that is named,
holds its Beauty for a short Time,
just for a moment before it dies.

IDEA ⇨ Intuition

With contemplation, a new Idea can rise, but this is only the beginning of the effort that needs to be undertaken. Permission needs to be given in order for the newness to find an efficient placement within some already accepted belief. The process of this placement, of giving the Idea a home, comes at a cost as it results in the Death of the Symbol, but also with a boon, the birth of an intuition.

Belief

Chooses comfort over conflict.

    Wears the costume of the staid.

Is just an effigy on the grave.

    Of what was thought of yesterday.

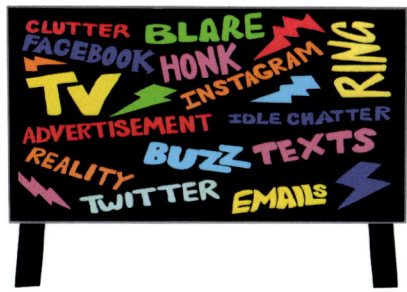

The quest for a perpetually conscious state,
dissembles its true motivation, which is the avoidance of
forgetfulness as it is understood to be the failure to
remember the facts and the fear of the
being forgotten.

The rational veneer of our daily lives is lived within the confines of the common sense, the product of culture which is based on the statistical likelihood of sameness and the safety of predictability as a protection against the threat of the arrival of the unknown. The irruption of the inexplicable is received by modern civilization as something that can be handled by the will. With effort, even Death is thought to be avoidable. With that willful amnesia to the Truth, we insulate ourselves from our own Destinies, failing to break through the restrictive sheath of comfort and convenience that is civilization.

Belief is frozen in nostalgia

The shock to the Mind that this little creature brings sets the stage for an escape of pent up energy from beneath the thin veneer that is conscious thought into the gaping relaxation that is the realm of understanding.

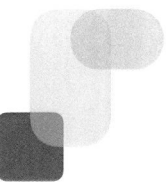

Culture, the sum total of the common sense of the masses, can be crushing and numbing to individuality. On some level, civilization holds the individual prisoner within its rigid structure of beliefs and mores. Culture has to be accepted as a tradeoff, that is to say, to gain protection one must give up autonomy. Without diligence, it is possible to lose track of one's Destiny.

The culture stands in for the conscious censor so that the sudden irruption of a too sudden change does not split the Mind and cause suffering. Suffering can be tolerated if it has been placed or grounded in a mythology that primes the Mind. If the story that sustains a people has died, the individual within a culture can lose orientation when there is no longer a sense of meaning. The mooring detaches and the Mind breaks away becoming uneasy with itself, adding "dis-ease" to the community.

The will believes in itself and when consciousness perceives itself to be failed by the will, the Mind turns to the manipulation of the natural world in an attempt to assuage the wound that impotence causes. Success in Life is a measurement, being a conscious construct, it is the causal aspect of the psychic event, a perception of control determined by the position of self relative to all things, even the subtle beings that populate the world.

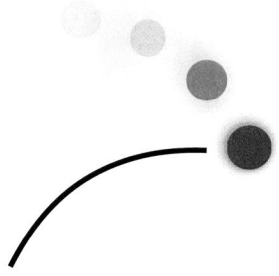

The unconscious is pointless without consciousness, as is
Reason meaningless without its grounding.

The ambit of consciousness may extend into the realm of understanding, which being characterized not only by the logic of Reason, but also by a depth of knowing, can be ambivalent, dynamic, and amplified through connection. In its most noble form, consciousness embraces the compassion that sees through the present and behind the past of memory and fantasy, bringing harmony with a shift in one's point of view away from self preoccupation to the concern for the other.

> With judgement, the more fascinating half of Life is thrown away.

Without having the language of the Heart to reach out to the Mind, the knowledge needed in the moment remains lost, unavailable to consciousness. Lost, but not quiet, resting in a shallow unmarked grave, it shifts erratically, moaning and groaning, causing dis-ease so that there is suffering. On some level, the Mind gets the message, but will it respond?

Culture, like the conscious censor,
protects the individual
from the shock of sudden change,
from the irruption of the unknown or unanticipated
that can be the source of suffering when the way of being
in the world is shallow.

Consciousness need not be limited to thought but may extend into the bailiwick of understanding. With understanding, the Mind releases its grasp on the buoys that are the small truths of daily Life, letting go of its obsession with facts. Sinking away from the surface, which is just the plot of Life, the Mind reaches the deeper currents of the motivation that runs behind thought.

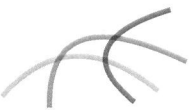

Until the strings are cut, the puppet is not truly free.

Words, once populated by the fragmented world of the pantheon, have become barren islands, literalized into signs without any depth to the message. Language must be allowed to come into consciousness pregnant with ambiguity, full of movement.

The curse in Life is to be mired in fixed remembrances,
in uprooted thought that has lost all connection to the Earth.

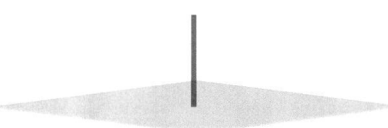

Eurydice is contentedly disconnected but in a way that is quite different from Orpheus who, cut off from his roots, from his Eurydice, stands less securely planted but all the more resolute for his ignorance.

Beneath Thought

The rhythm of the shaded place, like the candle in the cave,
runs behind the facts of Time like echoes from the grave.

Within the dark and damp of Her lies Wisdom as the Truth,
but in the glare of Him is naught but tragedy forsooth.

So be not fool, go guide the boat that rudderless, grounds near.
Take charge by letting go of thought and with it, all your fear.

To be civilized is to exist simply consciously in the world.

Uncertainty discombobulates consciousness.
Startled, we simply cannot center,
for the irrational has a shallow, broad field of focus.
It has no point of view while the rational sees only what it is focused upon.
It has but one focal point which is easily knocked askew.

Death

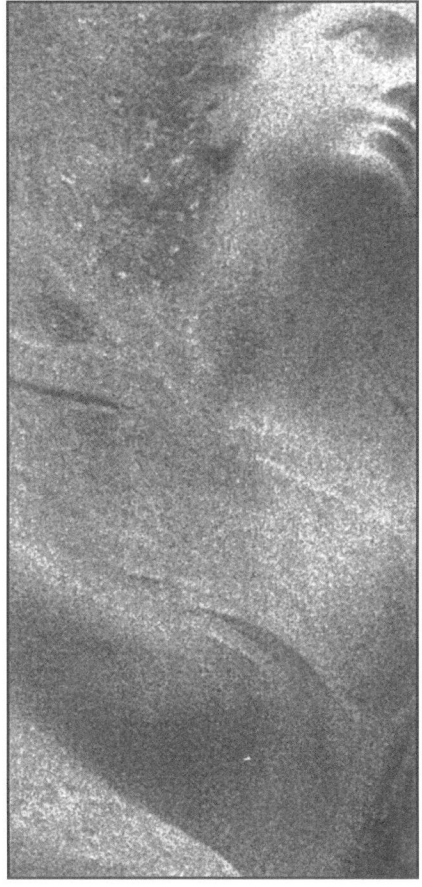

Life is wrapped in the arms of Death's tango.

Love makes Death personal in so many ways. Whether it is the arrival of a sense of absence with the first embrace, the separation from the body of a loved one through Death, the loss of the Beloved to the madness of the Mind, or perhaps most cruelly, abandonment by indifference, the passion of Love is always particular. Passionate love leaves as it comes, inexplicably. Even with compassion, we can relapse to the personal, to passion when loss pulls us out of balance and we fail to remember that in compassion all things remain.

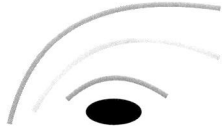

Fear separates us from the vastness of the Truth so that we remain in a state of psychic paralysis being too afraid to look Death in the face. We turn away from Nature and place plastic flowers and graven identities on resting places. The flowers remain, the identity stays, so where is Death? What does this say about our need to cling to the old belief, to deny Death a place in reality? This rote behavior may soothe the civilized Mind, it may quiet the anxiety of Reason, but it does not serve the dynamic between Spirit and Nature which is to bring into Life that which is outside of it, informing Life and giving Death its due place.

Lost in Space

Death is knowing what we forgot,
for in Life the memory fades,
save that moment or two when
we thought that we knew,
just before it all slipped away.

When the babe we still were,
the silver cord still in place,
there was a pulse that had its tide
within the flow of Divine grace.

Now cut off, the umbilicus dry,
tagged as members of the human race,
left suspended in the heaviness of Space,
we wait for our appointed escape.

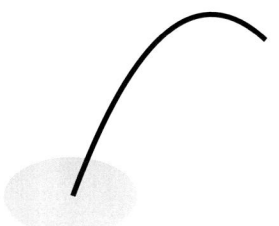

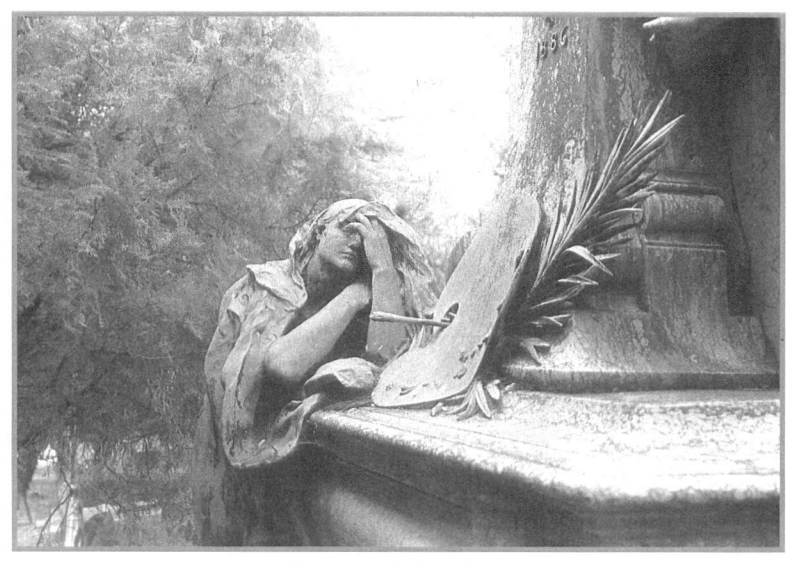

Père Lachaise, Paris

Death, set against the idea of Life is the root metaphor for all
the dynamics that lead to Knowing and to Being.
Love makes Death personal. As the scent of Love tarries,
the nauseatingly sweet odor of Death mingles.
It is the smell of the rose too long cut from the stem,
a sweet odor corrupted only by dread.

Sense of Absence

The pal that hangs in the air
when a Life has left
is like betrayal in Love
when the illusion shatters.

It is the sense of absence
as the connection is lost
and what was known
becomes what is forgot.

Death is a play populated by many actors,
a distant concern
until it is you who are beckoned to the stage.

The Gift of Death

Death, or the threat it, changes Life.
It brings a stinging meaning to it.
It is a gift that shocks the Mind into silence,
so Wisdom's voice may speak.

Death is the Space between the words
that the chattering Mind secretes,
a comma that forces thought to pause
so that Life takes Time to breathe.

Death evokes shapes of otherness
that once again or for the very first Time,
as non-local events at all points centered,
sync again with the internal rhyme.

Fear of Death paralyzes the Mind.

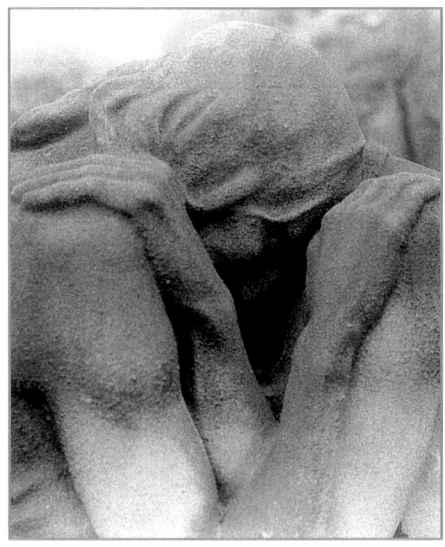

Père Lachaise, Paris

There is an oft traveled bridge from here to there
   Sometimes labeled Death, sometimes Love
      Made of loosened cobblestones
     That unsteady the gait of intention.

Love Makes Death Personal

Love makes Death personal
as does Death make Love Divine,
for the scent of Love does tarry
like the sweet sting of the vine.

Which poisons logic so it falls
a victim to deceit,
and Love can have its way again,
playing out its own conceit.

Love will have its way it seems,
forcing Heart from hearth to seek
the untrod path of healing ways
its own Death to bespeak.

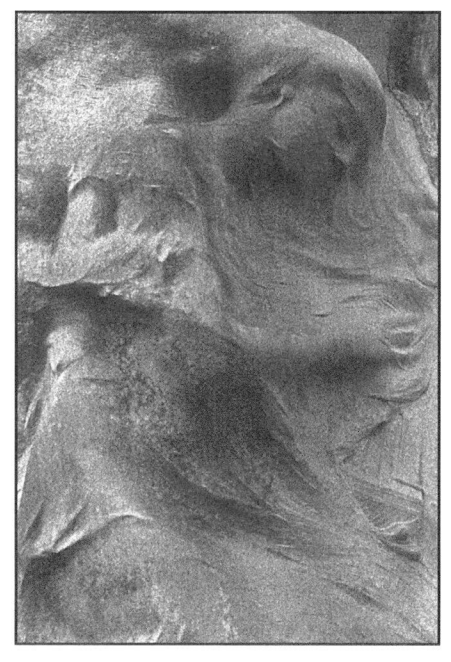

Death long ago begun
Just finished in this Dream
Of going down under
To swim in Nature's stream.

Death is the song that begins with the last breath of
Life.

Death considered consciously is usually limited to its literal meaning as the cessation of the Life of the Body, but when the Idea of Death is widened and deepened to its Image, it is the root metaphor for change. It might be helpful for those who find it hard to reflect on the Death of someone whom they loved to consider that rather than Death bringing the end to Life, Life exists within Death. In this way, one could take Life to be a moment within an Eternal Death. It is St. Augustine's perspective of the Divine, as whenever Time, Eternity.

The present moment is formed of the past as memory
and the future as Dream.
Awareness of the moment is *ab aeterno,* the gift of Death
as intuition.

Death is after all inclusive; it concerns everyone and is therefore a universal Truth. Life is the particular, the personal, an event and it needs to be deepened into an experience, which has to do with embracing Death. The experience of the Divine has to do with having the capacity to understand the role of Death in Life, one might say the skill to grasp the Truth of the Nature of things.

Love weaves Death into the fabric of the Mind.

Wisdom

Just as Life can see the moment
Death knows more than can be seen,
adding shadows to the sunlight
with what is garnered from the Dream.

The Void that Siphons

j

Death Too Early

We stutter, spinning in shock with the sudden change that is the
departure of the loved one.
Caught in a vortex, we become vertiginous,
disoriented.
For the too early Death is too much for the Mind to bear.

With the older ones,
there is an expectation of Death in Time.
There is a rhythm to being human that we accept.
But in the kidnapping of the young,
Reason cannot deal with the illogicality.

Reason Needs Conversation

Reason needs a conversation, but the silence that comes
with the kidnapping of the young ones, leaves Reason with no
Dream for company.

For Reason works out its reality in relationship to its Dreams.
During the night, each piece of the day
is placed in the cubby hole of meaning that is its proper place.

With the Death of the baby, order is disrupted,
Time looses its pace,
and the field of the Dream becomes overgrown with Space.

For the Death come too early
there is no lacunae that can be found
to place the darkness of the scene
in more familiar ground.

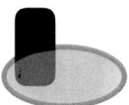

The River's Edge

I come to the edge of the River
to gain from this natural place.
It was here that my Dream first came to me,
and it is here that my Destiny awaits.

I come to the edge of the River
each year on this holy day,
the day they both chose to leave me,
the day we share this way.

I come to the edge of the River
to nurture this memory of mine,
grown so thin it can barely tote
its load of remembered Time.

I come to the edge of the River
for strength to suffer the weight,
of the one who left me too quickly,
of the other now meeting his fate.

So to the River's edge I've come
gently easing one to his grave
while reaching out for the other,
his place in my Life to save.

The Hands of Elizabeth

Her hands move more slowly,
her rhythm has changed,
for Time has no hold over them now.

The combatants are gone,
the battle is all done. All that remains is
silence and loss.

Elizabeth washes him gently,
changing the sheets back to white,
effacing all the stains of science.

Her hands carefully remove the tape,
the tubes and the synthetic things,
so the patient may again become babe.

As the restraints are released,
his body slumps naturally down,
as she cradles him in her hands.

Her loving fingertips follow the
curves of her little doll, and for the
first Time, her skin touches his.

She rubs the warmed baby oil
into the grayness of his skin,
so that a hint of Life might return.

She talks to him gently,
privately in the moment that she has
before she has to give him away.

Then the little suit comes out,
and the blanket that Grandma made.
Elizabeth covers him,
all but his sleeping face.

She gives him to his mother's arms
then turns to move away.
Even though her hands let go,
her heart will always stay.

Civilized Heart

The Death come too early is the boon
that is too great to bear
for the rootless Mind
ruled by a civilized Heart.

The too early Death wounds the Heart, leaving the Mind in stasis
and Reason in flight.

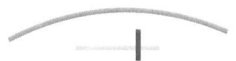

Divinity is not outside of any being. On the contrary…
they may be ignorant thereof. This happens because they
are fugitives…wandering outside of themselves.
(Plotinus VI.9)

The dead have a appetite for presence,
this is the Wisdom of Nature
wishing to be understood consciously.
With intuition there comes a shift in awareness,
and with that a momentary satiation of the thirst.

Truly Dead

To fail to grieve, leaves the dead undead.
When truly dead they can come within.
While without they remain un-grieved for.

As with our own mortality,
which when we fail to embrace it,
leaves us in Life the walking undead
rather than the truly alive.

So the premie,
who is too early to be reasonably alive,
is unreasonably undead, its "as if " status
leaving it outside, fluttering.

The Sandy Shore

Life is lived on the sandy shore,
while in the deep the serpents troll.
Her wetness swirls around us,
yet on dryness do we stroll.

Life lived within desiccation
is a series of arid events
that leaves us free from gravitas
but energy still spent…

Spent on endless rumination,
so that alive we are not,
somewhat dead but not dead enough,
the Vision yet forgot.

Destiny

Fallen Angel

Fallen Angel with no shadow
Flew too close to evade its plight
Lies before us outlined dimly
In rare flickers of Divine light.

As a candle follows its own thread
to an endpoint in the flame,
so the babe is consumed by Time,
given so few moments to remain.

Just a thin veneer protects it
and with Time it's peeled away
revealing what had lain well hidden,
within Destiny's shadow play.

The rooted Body is the repository of the Nature of Being. It is both genetic as an Aristotelean idea, an unfolding of predetermination, and epigenetic, a continuing process of modification and growth that echos the dialectic of Socrates. Both ways of genetic determination work together under the guise of Destiny engendering Life.

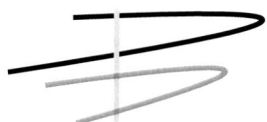

Destiny is the motivation behind the creation of Life.

"Then, after having sufficiently dwelt with it, she will, if she can, come to reveal to others this heavenly communion."

(Plotinus VI.9)

Divine

"for Divinity consists of being attached to the Center…"
(Plotinus VI.9)

The Divine fills the rearview of the Angel.

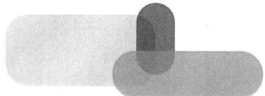

We teem with an ineffable longing when we catch a glimpse of the Divine. It triggers an anamnesis of the source of the spark and a desire to return to the whole.

The Divine is not limited to Time ,
but it is encumbered by it,
extending more freely into the realm of Death.

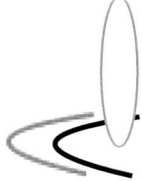

One cannot hear the prayer of the silent one,
the commune between the Angel and the babe.
One does not see it as a theophany,
a manifestation of the Divine in Time.

Doubt

Doubt is a method of knowing,
just as knowing is a doubtful way
of being in the world consciously,
all rigid stances to inveigh.

Doubt wedges itself between
what is known and what is not,
severing the connection
with a quick slice through the knot…

that kept them tethered to each other,
that kept the distance fixed,
between what was and what could well be,
the just orphaned and betwixt.

So the secret planted deeply,
the totality of what was known,
with the probe of doubt's intrusion
becomes the seed of intuition sown.

Doubt is a method of gaining knowledge.
It initiates the twist, the corkscrew movement
that pulls one down deeper into the matte of
one's blood-soaked roots.

Doubt initiates the decision to challenge
the status quo.

◇

Truth lies beneath the skin of the question.

●

Doubt, the willful bastard child of Reason
isolates thought, stranding the orphan who will have to
be searched for and carried back home.

Doubt is born of boredom with the singleminded preoccupation with history. It revives the personal and cultural myth with amusements from the imagination.

Doubt is necessary to prune the dry, dead branches that are one's personal half-truths, leaving room for native shoots to grow.

Doubt is the by-product of staleness,
the emission of
something that has overstayed its Time.

Death orphans the Mind from the Heart.
It wedges itself between them creating doubt
through disorientation. All that was fixed seems to break
away. All that was understood is thrown into question.
There is no safe harbor, for all
moorings have been ruptured.

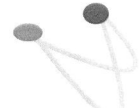

It is in the moment of doubt-driven confrontation during the turn away from the clarity of color and toward the ambiguity of gray, that thought as remembrance begins its transformation into Image. Through an internal rotation that realigns the psyche within itself, which is the process of mourning, one lets go of the idea of something. One lets slip the tight grasp of willful attachment and opens the Heart to the return of something new, the orphan re-envisioned.

Angels and Dreams

In Life, there is memory and there is forgetfulness. Outside of Life, there are the Angels whose Nature is such that they do not limit themselves to the either/or realism of manifestation. The Angel, being both literal and figurative, springs from the deep well which cannot be sounded. It is seemingly autonomous, self-feeding in that it creates the experience of its own event. It is beyond the control of consciousness as it reaches behind memory to recover the forgotten, not only the thought that lies buried beneath the gravestone, but the Wisdom that has yet to be remembered. The Angel reaches down for the Dream, for a version of the Original Vision, which as it rises to the surface, is transformed by the conscious censor into a form that Reason can fathom. With this, Reality shifts as Wisdom steps into the ever expanding landscape that is consciousness.

The Angel tutors the mind in unpleasant Truths as it whips up the landscape with the breeze from its wings, flying between the world as sensed and the world as intuited.

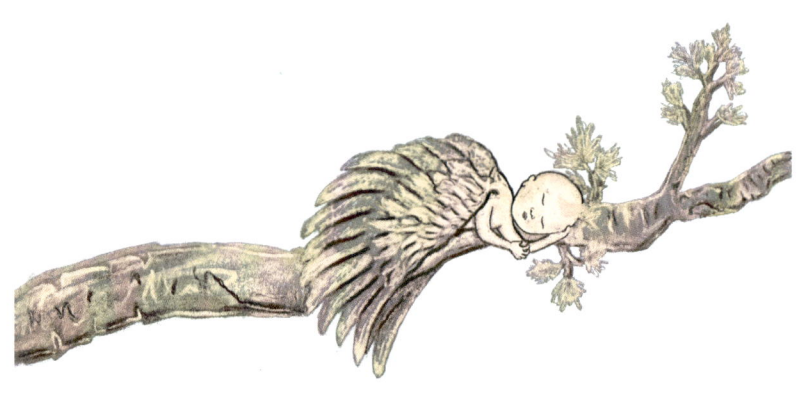

The Angel pulls us into the Dream as the Mind brushes the face of Eternity with its gaze.

The Dream

The tiny Life pulls one's attention.
The Mind goes to sleep and the imagination comes out to play
as the Dream comes to Life in the absence
of thought.

Whether it is approached as Freud's tangled web within which the rational is caught, wrapped in the repulsive, or Jung's natural realm, draped in a logic that attracts the attention of the conscious Mind, the Dream is imbedded, like the Symbol, with the power to direct energy. In the Dream rests the message of the objective realm as it rises into consciousness. The craving of the unknown to be known will out in spite of the willful repression of its contents, for the Dream will over Time finally reveal its secrets.

Just as light is not seen but generates sight, the Dream is not understood, but gives rise to insight.

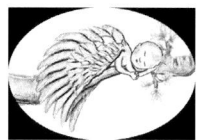

By working to develop a continually renewed and deepened brand of consciousness, the Dream when it is allowed to be real on its own terms, becomes the wonder of many ways. One way is not enough. One way is belief, the already seen, the too well known, the easily accepted that is tucked neatly into place.

The Dream is a conspiracy whose subversive action undermines both the authority of Reason and the autonomy of Nature, grafting one onto the other, so that what is imagined has both the mark of Eternity and the stamp of Time upon it.

Resistance to the Dream, reluctance to take it seriously, is the tendency of the modern individual. This misoneism, this fear of the unknown and of the new, is a product of willful reluctance by the conscious Mind to relinquish agency.

The Angel is not limited to the cyclical rumination of
everyday Life, just as the Dream stands outside of the
rhythm of Time and Space. The Angel roams in the landscape of the Dream,
surrounded by the dried roots of forgotten thoughts and the
tender plumules of tomorrow's intuitions.

A Deep Deep Sleep

I fell into a deep deep sleep
After days and days of tears
And what I dreamed, I dreamed so hard
Just to keep my memories near.

It was a dream of light and sight
A dream of sun and field
Of children playing in the grass
Their joy released in squeals.

A dream chock full of images
Children born, not of the flesh
Floating weightless as remembrances
By a silent, empty creche.

I slip into my Dream to find the river of my Life.

A Dream is born of the impulse to heal.
It is the incubator of the innovation that is meant
to rescue the culture from its lethargy, one Destiny at
a Time.

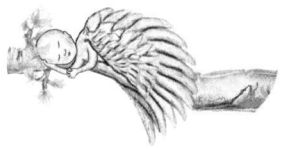

Dream is the taste of night left on the tongue of day.

Within the Dream, there is a sprouting of the original seed into
Time, of the universal then into the personal, as the unconscious is
directed toward the beaches of the islands of thought.

Dream plays out in a place that is not civilized, in the realm between Spirit and Nature. The Dream needs to be nurtured, not repressed, not dismissed, not laughed away. For being more than just the reflux of psychic indigestion, Dreams are the bittersweet remedy agains the acid of actuality.

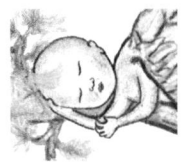

In the Wake of the Dream

Diminishing to its vanishing point,
the Dream with the morn will fade
yet the eye of the Mind in the wake of it
will replay its retinal display.

I Crawl Into My Dream

I crawl into my dream to sleep
For there my fantasies live
There I am loved, I think
There I am real, I think.

Here it is thick, I sense
All that I long for is just out of reach
All that I think I have, I cannot find
All that I think I need, eludes me.

I crawl into my dream with ease
For it is the place I need to be
Taking the space I need to see
Escaping the lights that glare at me.

With silence now in the dark of me
My hands hover over each black key
Of my little Mind machine that
Will click me away from here.

Duality-Tension

Affinity as the third thing defines all relationships,
tension and reconciliation,
conservation and progression.

The dipole reconciles to a greater power.

Within the tension that supports the psychic paradox, both consciousness, with its conservative stance and unconsciousness, as a progressive fluidity, are served. When the distance is reduced briefly by the power of the third thing, a reconciliation of the two perspectives of the Mind is accomplished resulting a new world view.

Like a Pendulum, Swing

Stay suspended in Life in such a way
that like the pendulum you swing
between the sides of any issue being raised.

Leap from stone to stone, cresting in midair,
assessing not one but all views at hand,
and never, never choose... only add.

Remain between knowing and understanding,
hanging between them like a counterweight,
relating loosely to all perspectives.

In this way, you stay awake.

The relationship that exists between any two things, affinity or the third thing, is what sets the perspective of the psyche above those of consciousness and unconsciousness which as independently functioning ways of being in and knowing the world, do not extend into the realm of becoming. The third thing reconciles the duality. The Angelic movement of the Spirit, the power of Compassion, and the Descent to Nature all address both the tension held and the temporary resolution of it. This relaxation of or loss of tension allows the rise of the orphaned knowledge as an intuition that becomes an aspect of the expanding consciousness leading the individual towards her/his path of Destiny and the culture towards its rescue.

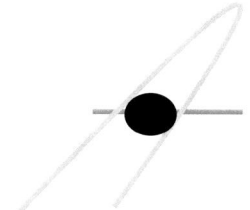

Event/Experience

We are in the end only events wishing to
experience themselves.

●

Life happens as an event
that is interned within a common sense. When it is
transformed
within the movement of Love, it
becomes a shared experience.

Thought Forgotten

While the event lives in thought
The experience does not
Being more than just fact
It will n'er be forgot.

For what is believed forgotten
In Truth lingers on
Secreted deep within lacunae
Revealed in Nature's spawn.

Fear

To be freed from fear is to be liberated from the mental paralysis of the one-perspective Life. The single perspective, the principle that has overstayed its usefulness is the dead myth, no longer vital to the individual psyche or the cultural health.

Fear comes from the failure to experience more than the common sense of things, which as the sum total of cultural mores and beliefs, tends to isolate one from the fullness of the Truth.

One has the choice not to remain ignorant, lingering in the comfort zone, holding on for dear Life to the cultural mainstays. That is the fate of civilized consciousness, the tattered edges of its thoughts caught in a net of fear. Cut loose from the net, release the tension, refresh the myth, and live.

Idea/Eidos

The Angel, is the Greek *eidos,*
both the thing and the means to it.
She is self-feeding, the Idea that leads to itself,
building up a storehouse of
experience.

Healing

Wishing to know more deeply, the Spirit, which as the spark of the Divine, probes beyond the literal of *logos* to the gestural of *mythos* in order to find the story behind the facts, shelling the event to find its pearl.

By eschewing belief for the Truth, letting go of the addiction to expectation, the Mind discovers the other half of itself, the source of all of its experience. It finds the reservoir of meaning, the hollow of Dream seeds within the depths of its own Being.

Finding the deeper way of knowing, consciousness adds understanding to intellect, leaving the isolation of the single perspective behind in a turn back to Nature. In this way, the Mind rediscovers the Truth that is native to it.

> We are but salt dolls soon to return to the sea.

Reference for Plotinus quotes

Guthrie, Kenneth Sylvan. 2017. *Plotinus Complete Works.* Kshetra Books (89-91).

Postface

Healing is the action of opening to the other; it becomes possible within a state of Mind that encourages inclusion rather than exclusion, allowing an occupation as the natural moves into thought as the Truth.

The experience of the too early born is an angelic movement by which we can be occupied by the Truth. I have written these books, *A Fate Unwound Too Soon* and its companion books, in the hope that they will serve to evoke the meaning necessary to make the experience of reading them a means to reveal some part of the secret that for too long and far too often has remained concealed.